RITUAL ESSENTIAL FOR WOMEN PRENATAL GUIDE

Your Essential Path to a Healthy

Nourishing Pregnancy

Dr. Anna A. Mejia

Copyright © 2024 by Dr. Anna A. Mejia

All rights reserved. No part of this publication may be reproduced, distributed, or transmitted in any form or by any means, including photocopying, recording, or other electronic or mechanical methods, without the prior written permission of the publisher, except in the case of brief quotations embodied in critical reviews and certain other noncommercial uses permitted by copyright.

TABLE OF CONTENT

- INTRODUCTION
- CHAPTER 1: UNDERSTANDING RITUAL ESSENTIAL PRENATAL MULTIVITAMIN
- CHAPTER 2: NUTRITIONAL PROFILE OF RITUAL PRENATAL
- CHAPTER 3: HOW TO TAKE RITUAL PRENATAL MULTIVITAMIN
- CHAPTER 4: ADMINISTRATION AND FORMULATION
- CHAPTER 5. POTENTIAL SIDE EFFECTS AND HOW TO MANAGE THEM
- CHAPTER 6: PRECAUTIONS AND CONTRAINDICATIONS
- CHAPTER 7: EXPECTED BENEFITS OF RITUAL PRENATAL MULTIVITAMIN
- CHAPTER 8: INTERACTIONS WITH OTHER SUPPLEMENTS AND MEDICATIONS
- CHAPTER 9: STORAGE AND HANDLING OF RITUAL PRENATAL
- CHAPTER 10: FREQUENTLY ASKED QUESTIONS
- CONCLUSION

INTRODUCTION

Pregnancy is an incredible journey, filled with excitement, anticipation, and countless choices that shape the health and well-being of both mother and baby. One of the most essential decisions is ensuring the right nutrients are consistently available to support your growing baby's development.

Ritual Essential for Women Prenatal Multivitamin with Folate & Choline is crafted to meet these needs in a modern, scientifically-backed way, offering a blend of carefully selected nutrients that play a vital role in pregnancy. In this guide, we dive into what makes Ritual Prenatal Multivitamin a powerful choice for expecting mothers, providing a straightforward roadmap to using it effectively. Every expectant mother deserves to feel confident in her prenatal choices, and with the complexities of modern-day supplements, understanding why certain ingredients matter is key to taking charge of prenatal health.

Ritual's Prenatal Multivitamin is more than just a daily pill—it's a blend of purposeful nutrients that align with your body's unique requirements during pregnancy. For example, the addition of folate and choline, two often overlooked nutrients, provides targeted support in ways other multivitamins can sometimes miss. Folate is essential for healthy cell growth, especially for your baby's neural tube development in the early stages of pregnancy, which becomes the brain and spinal cord.

Meanwhile, choline supports fetal brain development and may contribute to lifelong cognitive health. Together, these nutrients build a strong foundation for your baby's development, while also ensuring you're supported physically, as well. Yet, what truly sets Ritual's Prenatal Multivitamin apart is its commitment to quality and transparency. In a world where so many products are available, it's easy to become overwhelmed. Ritual aims to simplify this by making every ingredient traceable. The brand provides transparency down to the source of each nutrient, so you know exactly where each part of the supplement originates.

Additionally, each bottle goes through rigorous third-party testing for purity and potency, meaning you can trust that what's on the label is exactly what you're putting into your body. The capsules themselves are designed for convenience and ease of use. They are encapsulated with delayed-release technology, which means the nutrients are absorbed gradually, minimizing any chance of stomach upset—a welcome feature for many expecting mothers who deal with morning sickness and digestive sensitivity.

On top of this, Ritual has added a pleasant lemon essence tab to each capsule, which helps mask the typical aftertaste of a multivitamin and makes it easier to consume daily. As important as the ingredients themselves are, taking a prenatal multivitamin shouldn't be overwhelming or inconvenient. Ritual understands the lifestyle of modern moms-to-be and offers a subscription-based delivery system. This setup guarantees that you never miss a dose simply because you ran out.

Instead, the supplements are delivered to your door each month, eliminating one more thing to worry about. For moms who are always on the go or adjusting to life with pregnancy, this consistent availability can make a significant difference in staying on track with prenatal health. But as with any supplement, understanding the potential effects, both positive and negative, is essential. While Ritual Essential Prenatal is designed to be well-tolerated, some women may experience mild digestive side effects or what's often referred to as "fishy burps" due to the omega-3 content.

Knowing what to expect and how to adjust can make all the difference in maintaining a comfortable and beneficial routine. Later in this guide, we'll cover strategies to manage any mild side effects and tips to get the most from each dose, ensuring it aligns with your body's natural rhythms. This guide will also explore how Ritual's prenatal vitamins compare to other options on the market. Every pregnancy journey is unique, and while Ritual offers a powerful blend of core nutrients, it's essential to understand how it fits within the broader landscape of prenatal supplements. For some women, it might be the perfect standalone option, while others may choose to add complementary nutrients based on personal needs and medical advice. Ultimately, Ritual Essential Prenatal Multivitamin is more than a supplement; it's a choice rooted in science, designed to meet the specific needs of the modern, mindful mother. It's for women who prioritize their health and well-being, who value transparency in what they consume, and who are committed to giving their baby the very best start in life.

The ritual of taking a prenatal vitamin daily is simple but incredibly meaningful. With each capsule, you're investing in the health of both yourself and your child. As we dive deeper into this guide, our aim is to provide you with clear, practical information on every aspect of Ritual Prenatal Multivitamin: how to take it, when to take it, and what to expect. We'll discuss each nutrient, explain the science behind it, and give you tips on how to maximize its benefits.

Whether this is your first pregnancy or an addition to a growing family, this guide is here to help you feel empowered in making the best choices for your prenatal health. Motherhood starts long before the baby arrives, and taking a daily prenatal vitamin like Ritual is one of the simplest, most impactful ways to nourish both you and your baby from the very beginning.

CHAPTER 1; UNDERSTANDING RITUAL ESSENTIAL PRENATAL MULTIVITAMIN

Overview of the Product

Ritual Essential for Women Prenatal Multivitamin is a thoughtfully crafted dietary supplement designed to support the unique nutritional needs of women during pregnancy. As a time of remarkable change, pregnancy requires a heightened focus on nutrition, making it vital for expectant mothers to consider their vitamin and mineral intake. Ritual recognizes this need and offers a product that not only meets these requirements but does so with transparency and quality. Each bottle of Ritual Prenatal Multivitamin contains a blend of essential nutrients tailored to promote the health of both mother and baby. Unlike many traditional prenatal vitamins that can be overwhelming in their ingredient lists and often contain additives or fillers, Ritual focuses on simplicity and effectiveness.

The product is designed to be easy to digest, featuring a delayed-release capsule that ensures the vitamins are absorbed efficiently in the small intestine, where nutrient absorption is optimal. What sets Ritual apart is its commitment to ingredient transparency. Each nutrient is sourced with care, and the company provides detailed information about the origins of each ingredient. This commitment to quality means that users can trust what they are consuming and feel confident that they are providing their bodies with the best possible support during this critical time.

Purpose and Target Audience

The primary purpose of Ritual Essential Prenatal Multivitamin is to fill the nutritional gaps that may arise during pregnancy. Pregnancy places unique demands on a woman's body, requiring additional vitamins and minerals to support the developing fetus. The target audience for this product includes expectant mothers who want to ensure they are meeting their nutritional needs while also promoting the health and development of their baby. Understanding the needs of pregnant women, Ritual designed this multivitamin to be suitable for those who might struggle with conventional prenatal vitamins due to their taste, size, or the gastrointestinal discomfort they can sometimes cause. By providing a product that is free from sugar, gluten, dairy, and artificial additives, Ritual appeals to a wide audience, including those with dietary restrictions or sensitivities.

Moreover, Ritual recognizes that the journey to motherhood often begins before conception. Many women seek to improve their health and nutritional intake in preparation for pregnancy. As such, this multivitamin can also be a proactive choice for women planning to conceive, ensuring that their bodies are well-equipped with the essential nutrients needed for a healthy pregnancy.

Key Ingredients and Nutritional Benefits

At the heart of Ritual Essential Prenatal Multivitamin are several key ingredients that play crucial roles in maternal and fetal health. Let's explore these components and their respective benefits:

1. Folate (800 mcg): Folate is one of the most critical nutrients for pregnant women, as it helps prevent neural tube defects, which can affect the brain and spinal cord. It is essential for DNA synthesis and cell growth, making it vital during the early stages of pregnancy when the fetal neural tube is forming. Ritual uses a bioavailable form of folate, methylfolate, which is easier for the body to absorb.

2. Choline (55 mg): Often overshadowed by other nutrients, choline is crucial for brain development and function. It supports the formation of neurotransmitters, which are essential for communication within the brain. Adequate choline intake during pregnancy is associated

with improved cognitive outcomes for the child. Ritual includes this important nutrient to ensure mothers have enough for both their health and their baby's development.

3. Iron (30 mg): Iron is essential for producing hemoglobin, the protein in red blood cells that carries oxygen throughout the body. During pregnancy, a woman's blood volume increases significantly, leading to a higher demand for iron. Sufficient iron intake helps prevent anemia, which can cause fatigue and other health issues.

4. Vitamin D (600 IU): Vitamin D is crucial for calcium absorption and plays a significant role in bone health. It supports the immune system and is believed to have a positive impact on mood. Adequate vitamin D levels are essential during pregnancy to ensure proper fetal development, especially regarding bone growth and overall health.

5. Omega-3 Fatty Acids (DHA): These healthy fats are vital for brain and eye development in the fetus. DHA is linked to improved cognitive function and visual acuity in infants. While many prenatal vitamins do not include omega-3s, Ritual recognizes their importance and incorporates them into their formula for added support.

6. Iodine (150 mcg): Iodine is necessary for healthy thyroid function, which regulates metabolism and is crucial for fetal brain development. During pregnancy, the demand for iodine increases, making it essential to ensure adequate intake to support both the mother's and the baby's health.

7. Vitamin B12 (2.6 mcg): This vitamin is vital for energy production, neurological function, and the formation of red blood cells. For vegetarians and vegans, who may struggle to obtain sufficient B12 from food sources, Ritual offers an important supplementation option to ensure this nutrient is adequately supplied.

Ritual Essential Prenatal Multivitamin stands out not only for its carefully selected ingredients but also for its formulation that addresses common concerns associated with prenatal vitamins. The use of a delayed-release capsule minimizes stomach upset, making it easier for mothers to take daily without discomfort.

In summary, Ritual Essential Prenatal Multivitamin is more than just a supplement; it's a carefully crafted blend of essential nutrients designed to support the health of both mothers and their developing babies. With its commitment to transparency, quality, and ease of use, it stands as an excellent choice for expectant mothers seeking a reliable prenatal multivitamin. As we continue to explore this guide, we'll delve into how to properly use this product, what to expect, and how to maximize its benefits for a healthy pregnancy.

CHAPTER 2: NUTRITIONAL PROFILE OF RITUAL PRENATAL

As we journey further into understanding Ritual Essential Prenatal Multivitamin, it's crucial to dive into its nutritional profile. Pregnancy is a phase where every nutrient counts, impacting both the mother's health and the baby's development. The ingredients in Ritual Prenatal are purposefully selected to offer comprehensive support during this vital time, filling nutritional gaps that can arise even with a balanced diet. In this chapter, we'll take a closer look at the detailed composition of this multivitamin, analyze each ingredient, and explain how these nutrients contribute to the well-being of both mother and baby.

Detailed Ingredient Analysis

Ritual Prenatal Multivitamin sets itself apart by emphasizing ingredient transparency and purity, offering a clean formulation without unnecessary fillers, artificial colorants, or additives. Each nutrient included in Ritual Prenatal serves a specific function, ensuring that both the mother's health and the baby's development are supported optimally.

1. Folate (Methylated Form - 800 mcg)

Folate is one of the most critical nutrients during pregnancy, playing an essential role in cell division, DNA synthesis, and neural tube formation in the fetus. Ritual uses the methylated form of folate, known as methylfolate, which is more bioavailable and easily absorbed by the body, compared to the synthetic form, folic acid. This nutrient helps prevent neural tube defects, making it a vital component in prenatal health.

2. Choline (55 mg)

Choline, though not as commonly highlighted as other nutrients, is critical for brain and cognitive development. It aids in the formation of cell membranes and supports the development of the spinal cord and brain in the fetus. Choline is essential for expectant mothers, as it also aids in liver function and reduces the risk of neural tube defects, making it a powerful ally for both mother and baby.

3. Iron (30 mg)

Pregnancy often increases a woman's blood volume by 50%, which can put a strain on iron reserves. Iron is necessary for the production of hemoglobin, the protein that helps transport oxygen throughout the body. Ritual's dose of 30 mg helps reduce the risk of anemia, supports the mother's increased blood production needs, and delivers oxygen efficiently to the developing baby.

4. Vitamin D (600 IU)

Vitamin D is indispensable for calcium absorption, bone health, and immune support. During pregnancy, it supports the development of the fetal skeleton and reduces the risk of preterm birth. Ritual includes 600 IU of vitamin D, an amount that aligns with recommended intake levels to support both mother and baby.

5. Omega-3 DHA (200 mg)

Omega-3 fatty acids, specifically DHA, play a significant role in fetal brain and eye development. Ritual includes 200 mg of DHA sourced from microalgae, making it a sustainable, plant-based option, and an excellent choice for vegetarians and vegans. This DHA is critical during the later stages of pregnancy when the baby's brain is rapidly growing and developing.

6. Iodine (150 mcg)

Iodine is essential for healthy thyroid function, which regulates metabolism and is key to neurological development in the fetus. During pregnancy, the thyroid hormone needs increase, making iodine crucial to prevent developmental issues in the baby and support the mother's thyroid health.

7. Vitamin B12 (2.8 mcg)

Vitamin B12 is necessary for the production of red blood cells, DNA synthesis, and neurological function. It's especially important for women who follow a vegetarian or vegan diet, as it is commonly found in animal products. Including B12 in Ritual's formula helps prevent deficiency and supports energy levels and nerve health.

8. Magnesium (30 mg)

Magnesium aids in muscle relaxation, reduces the risk of leg cramps, and helps regulate blood pressure. For expectant mothers, it can also play a role in promoting calm and better sleep, which are both essential for physical and mental well-being during pregnancy.

Role of Folate, Choline, and Other Essential Nutrients

Each nutrient in Ritual Prenatal is included for its critical role in maternal and fetal health:

Folate and Choline are champions in early fetal development, crucial for forming the brain and spinal cord. Folate's role in DNA synthesis and neural tube formation makes it vital during the first trimester, while choline supports cognitive health and brain function.

Iron and Vitamin B12 work together to support oxygen transport and energy production. Iron is the foundation for blood production, while B12 supports healthy red blood cells, reducing the likelihood of fatigue and anemia.

Vitamin D and Magnesium play interconnected roles in bone health. While vitamin D enhances calcium absorption for skeletal development, magnesium aids in nerve function and reduces muscle cramps, which are common discomforts during pregnancy.

Omega-3 DHA supports brain and eye development. Including DHA from microalgae aligns with Ritual's commitment to sustainability and vegetarian-friendly sourcing. Omega-3s are essential during the final trimester when the baby's brain is developing at a rapid pace.

Nutritional Benefits for Mother and Baby

Ritual's carefully chosen nutrients offer multi-faceted benefits, fostering a healthy pregnancy for both mother and child. For mothers, these vitamins and minerals fill potential dietary gaps, support increased blood volume, help with energy production, and promote mental clarity. This balanced nutritional profile is tailored to ease common pregnancy symptoms, such as fatigue, nausea, and leg cramps, while enhancing overall well-being.

For the developing baby, the benefits are foundational and long-lasting. Folate and choline support neural development, helping establish a solid cognitive base. DHA and iodine contribute to brain function and neurological development, fostering optimal mental and physical growth. Iron and B12 ensure the baby receives adequate oxygen for growth, while magnesium and vitamin D build a strong skeletal structure.

Furthermore, the quality and bioavailability of these ingredients ensure that the mother's body can effectively absorb and utilize each nutrient. Ritual's transparency in sourcing, and commitment to clean, non-GMO ingredients, ensures that expectant mothers can trust what they're taking, providing peace of mind during a pivotal time.

In essence, Ritual Essential Prenatal Multivitamin's nutritional profile stands as a testament to the importance of well-rounded prenatal care. With its precise blend of essential nutrients, it is an invaluable ally for women aiming to nourish their bodies and nurture their babies from conception through pregnancy. This chapter only begins to explore the science behind these nutrients, setting the stage for understanding the broader impact of quality prenatal care in the chapters to come.

CHAPTER 3; HOW TO TAKE RITUAL PRENATAL MULTIVITAMIN

Taking a prenatal vitamin is one of the simplest ways to support a healthy pregnancy. But ensuring you're getting the maximum benefit from your supplement can sometimes feel overwhelming. In this chapter, we break down everything you need to know to make taking Ritual Essential Prenatal Multivitamin easy, effective, and adaptable to your unique needs. By understanding the right dosage, best practices for absorption, and ways to adjust your intake based on personal circumstances, you can confidently incorporate Ritual Prenatal into your daily routine.

Recommended Dosage and Timing

The recommended dosage for Ritual Prenatal Multivitamin is two capsules per day. This dosage has been carefully formulated to deliver the precise amount of essential nutrients needed during pregnancy, such as folate, choline, and iron, without the risk of overconsumption.

When to Take It

One of the best things about Ritual Prenatal is its flexible timing. You don't need to take it with food, thanks to its gentle formula and delayed-release capsules that dissolve in the small intestine rather than the stomach. This means you can incorporate it into your routine when it's most convenient for you. However, taking it at the same time each day can help build a habit, reducing the likelihood of forgetting. Whether you choose morning, midday, or evening, consistency is key.

Morning vs. Evening

Some women find that taking prenatal vitamins in the morning boosts their energy and starts their day off right, while others prefer taking them in the evening when they're winding down. If you experience mild nausea or digestive discomfort, evening might be the better option as it allows you to sleep through any mild side effects. Testing out different times of day can help you identify what feels best for you.

Directions for Best Absorption

To make the most of Ritual's carefully selected ingredients, it's essential to understand how best to promote absorption. The body's ability to absorb vitamins and minerals can vary based on several factors, including hydration levels, timing, and even other foods or supplements in your system.

Hydration and Water Intake
Taking Ritual Prenatal with a full glass of water is beneficial for several reasons. Water helps the capsules dissolve and pass through the digestive system more efficiently. Staying hydrated also promotes overall digestion, which can support absorption across the board. However, try to avoid excessive amounts of water

at once, as this can dilute stomach acids, potentially slowing down digestion.

Timing Around Meals

While Ritual Prenatal is gentle enough to take on an empty stomach, some vitamins—like fat-soluble vitamins A, D, E, and K—absorb better when taken with a source of healthy fat. If you have the option, try pairing your capsule with a snack or meal that contains a bit of healthy fat, like avocado, nuts, or yogurt. This can help maximize the benefits of the fat-soluble vitamins in the formula without causing any digestive strain.

Avoid Taking with Certain Foods or Beverages

Some substances can interfere with nutrient absorption, so it's helpful to be mindful of what you consume around the time you take your prenatal vitamin. For example, calcium can inhibit iron absorption, so it's a good idea to avoid taking Ritual Prenatal with a large amount of dairy. Similarly, beverages like coffee or tea contain compounds that can reduce the absorption of certain nutrients. If you love your morning coffee or tea, consider taking Ritual Prenatal either 1-2 hours before or after your caffeine fix to ensure you're not compromising any nutrient intake.

Situational Modifications

Every pregnancy is unique, and the ways you adapt your prenatal routine can make a difference in how you feel each day. Below are some common scenarios and modifications to help ensure that you're getting the most out of Ritual Prenatal, no matter your situation.

Morning Sickness

For many pregnant women, morning sickness can make it difficult to keep food and supplements down, especially during the first trimester. If you're struggling with nausea:

1. Take the Capsules at Night

Shifting your intake to the evening can help prevent the capsules from exacerbating any nausea you might experience in the morning. Many women find that symptoms ease as the day goes on, making it easier to keep their prenatal vitamins down in the evening.

2. Split the Dosage

If taking both capsules at once feels overwhelming, consider splitting the dose throughout the day. For example, you can take one capsule in the morning and one in the evening, reducing the likelihood of nausea while still getting the full daily dose.

3. Try with Bland Foods

If you find that taking the capsules with food eases your nausea, pair them with bland, easily digestible foods like toast or crackers. This provides a buffer for your stomach without triggering nausea.

Dietary Restrictions

Ritual Prenatal is designed to be allergen-friendly, free from gluten, dairy, nuts, and artificial additives, making it suitable for many different dietary preferences. However, specific diets or restrictions may still impact how and when you take your prenatal vitamin.

1. Vegetarian and Vegan Diets
Ritual Prenatal is vegan-friendly and provides omega-3 DHA from microalgae rather than fish, which aligns with a plant-based diet. It also includes a good amount of iron and vitamin B12, which are often challenging to obtain on a vegetarian or vegan diet. If you follow a plant-based diet, rest assured that Ritual Prenatal is already tailored to meet your needs without requiring further modification.

2. Low-Calorie or Intermittent Fasting
If you're following a specific eating schedule, such as intermittent fasting, take your Ritual Prenatal during

your eating window for optimal absorption, especially if you consume healthy fats during that time. Since Ritual is designed to be easy on an empty stomach, it won't disrupt your fasting period, but the absorption of fat-soluble vitamins may improve with food.

3. Sensitive to Iron

Some individuals experience mild constipation or digestive discomfort with iron. Ritual includes a gentle, stomach-friendly form of iron, but if you're still sensitive, ensure you're drinking plenty of water throughout the day and incorporating fiber-rich foods into your diet. If issues persist, speak with your healthcare provider about any further modifications.

High-Activity Levels

If you lead a very active lifestyle or are an athlete, your body's nutritional demands may be higher. Ritual Prenatal is designed to offer balanced support, but combining it with a nutrient-dense diet rich in protein, complex carbs, and healthy fats will best support both prenatal needs and physical activity. Try taking the capsules with a post-workout snack that includes healthy fats to ensure you're replenishing and absorbing nutrients effectively.

Incorporating Ritual Essential Prenatal into your daily routine doesn't have to be complicated. By following the recommended dosage, being mindful of timing for optimal absorption, and making simple adjustments based on your unique needs, you can ensure you're receiving the full spectrum of benefits this prenatal has to offer. Remember, consistency is key. Creating a habit that aligns with your lifestyle will make it easy to support your pregnancy journey every day. Each capsule is designed to fill crucial nutritional gaps and help you provide the best foundation for yourself and your growing baby.

CHAPTER 4; ADMINISTRATION AND FORMULATION

Ritual Essential Prenatal Multivitamin stands out not only for its powerful nutrient blend but also for its innovative capsule design. Thoughtfully engineered to enhance ease of use, minimize nausea, and support optimal nutrient delivery, this multivitamin takes a modern approach to prenatal health. In this chapter, we'll explore the carefully designed features of Ritual's capsule, including its delayed-release technology and lemon-essenced flavor tabs, as well as tips to help you comfortably incorporate it into your routine without any discomfort.

Capsule Design and Delayed-Release Technology

The capsule of Ritual Essential Prenatal Multivitamin is as innovative as the nutrients inside. The outer shell of each capsule is designed with delayed-release technology—a feature that allows the capsule to dissolve in the small intestine rather than the stomach. This thoughtful design helps ensure that you receive the full benefit of each nutrient without common gastrointestinal side effects like nausea or stomach upset, which are often associated with traditional prenatal vitamins.

Benefits of Delayed-Release

The delayed-release mechanism provides several key advantages. Firstly, because the nutrients are absorbed in the small intestine rather than the stomach, they're processed at a more natural pace, allowing for better nutrient uptake. This also reduces the likelihood of stomach irritation, which is especially important for pregnant women who may already be dealing with symptoms like morning sickness. By bypassing the stomach's acidic environment, Ritual's delayed-release capsules can deliver sensitive nutrients—such as folate and omega-3s—more effectively and comfortably.

This technology is also particularly beneficial for essential nutrients that require gentle absorption, such as iron and folate. The stomach-friendly iron used in Ritual's formula is less likely to cause the digestive discomfort sometimes experienced with other iron supplements, making it easier to tolerate even for those with sensitive stomachs.

Transparency and Ingredient Quality
The design of the capsule also reflects Ritual's commitment to transparency. Ritual capsules are made from plant-based materials and contain no artificial additives, colors, or fillers, so you know exactly what you're putting into your body. Ritual goes the extra mile to ensure each ingredient is ethically sourced, vegan-friendly, and non-GMO. This integrity in sourcing, combined with the gentle delivery system, makes Ritual a trustworthy choice for pregnant women looking for effective, reliable nutrition.

Overview of Flavor Tabs (Lemon Essence)

Another unique aspect of Ritual Essential Prenatal Multivitamin is its lemon-essenced flavor tab. Traditional prenatal vitamins are often associated with unpleasant tastes or aftertastes, which can be especially off-putting when pregnant women are already dealing with food aversions and heightened senses. Ritual has addressed this by adding a subtle, refreshing lemon essence to each capsule.

Why Lemon Essence?
The lemon flavor tab serves multiple purposes beyond just taste. For one, citrus has natural anti-nausea properties, making it an ideal choice for a prenatal vitamin. Many pregnant women find that the lemon essence helps counteract any lingering vitamin aftertaste, making it easier and more enjoyable to take consistently. Additionally, the lemon essence is designed to provide a gentle, clean flavor that doesn't overwhelm or clash with other foods or beverages you might be consuming.

Unlike artificially flavored vitamins, which can sometimes taste overly sweet or harsh, Ritual's lemon essence is subtle, refreshing, and natural. The flavor is created using natural lemon oil, ensuring that even those with sensitive palates can appreciate it. The flavor tab is particularly helpful if you're taking the vitamin on an empty stomach, as it can offer a slight reprieve from the "vitamin taste" that some individuals experience. This touch of flavor doesn't alter the efficacy of the capsule but rather complements it, making your daily supplement routine smoother and more pleasant.

Recommendations for Swallowing and Avoiding Nausea

Taking pills can sometimes be challenging, especially if you're experiencing morning sickness or general nausea, which is common during pregnancy. Ritual has kept these challenges in mind by creating a prenatal that's easier to swallow, with additional tips for maximizing comfort.

Tips for Swallowing the Capsule

While Ritual capsules are standard in size, they are streamlined and designed with ease in mind. Here are some recommendations to make swallowing the capsule simpler:

1. Take with a Full Glass of Water
Drinking a full glass of water not only aids in swallowing but also helps the capsule move smoothly through the digestive tract. This also supports hydration, which is essential during pregnancy.

2. Pair with a Small Snack
Although Ritual Prenatal doesn't require food for proper absorption, if you're struggling with swallowing or mild nausea, pairing it with a bland snack, like crackers or applesauce, can ease the process.

3. Tilt Forward
While many people instinctively tilt their heads back when swallowing pills, tilting your head slightly forward

can actually help open the esophagus, making it easier to swallow.

Avoiding Nausea

Ritual Prenatal's gentle formulation and delayed-release technology are designed to be kind on the stomach, yet everyone's experience with prenatal vitamins can vary. If nausea is a concern, here are some strategies to help:

1. Take at Night

If you're prone to morning sickness, consider taking Ritual Prenatal in the evening. Many women find that nausea is less pronounced later in the day, making it easier to keep the vitamin down without discomfort.

2. Split the Dosage

While the recommended dosage is two capsules per day, you can take them separately—one in the morning and one in the evening—if you find it helps with nausea. This approach ensures that you're getting your daily intake without overwhelming your stomach.

3. Pair with Ginger or Lemon Tea

Both ginger and lemon have natural anti-nausea properties, which can be helpful if you're sensitive to vitamins. A cup of ginger tea or a squeeze of lemon in water can help ease nausea and make taking your prenatal vitamin more comfortable.

4. Try Breathing Techniques

If the mere thought of swallowing a pill triggers queasiness, a few calming breaths can help. Try taking a few deep breaths before and after swallowing to help calm your system and reduce any anticipatory nausea.

Establishing a Routine for Consistency

Consistency is key when it comes to prenatal vitamins. Creating a routine that aligns with your lifestyle and preferences can make it easier to remember to take your vitamins and help your body establish a rhythm for absorbing the nutrients.

1. Set a Daily Reminder

Use a phone alarm or an app to remind yourself each day. The easier you make it to remember, the more likely you'll stick with it.

2. Choose a Comfortable Location

Keep your Ritual Prenatal in a spot you associate with your daily routine, such as next to your toothbrush, on your nightstand, or in the kitchen near your morning coffee or tea. This visual cue can help prompt you to take it daily.

3. Incorporate Self-Care

Consider your prenatal vitamin as part of a self-care ritual. Pair it with a few moments of quiet, reflection, or relaxation to reinforce the idea that you're doing something positive for yourself and your baby. This intentional approach can turn taking your vitamin into something you look forward to rather than a chore.

Ritual Essential Prenatal Multivitamin isn't just a nutrient-dense supplement; it's a thoughtfully designed tool to support your pregnancy journey. With its delayed-release capsule, refreshing lemon essence, and flexibility for different personal needs, Ritual offers a prenatal vitamin that fits seamlessly into modern life. By following these tips and finding what works best for you, you can maximize your experience with Ritual Prenatal, making each dose a smooth and beneficial part of your day. Whether you're new to prenatals or seeking a more comfortable option, Ritual Prenatal innovative design and approachable format make it a valuable addition to your wellness routine.

CHAPTER 5. POTENTIAL SIDE EFFECTS AND HOW TO MANAGE THEM

When choosing a prenatal vitamin, understanding possible side effects and knowing how to manage them can make a world of difference in maintaining a healthy, comfortable experience. While Ritual Essential Prenatal Multivitamin is designed to be gentle and easy to digest, it's still a blend of potent nutrients that may, on occasion, cause minor discomfort as your body adjusts. This chapter covers common side effects like nausea and digestive changes, explores rare but possible reactions, and offers practical tips to minimize and manage these issues for a smoother journey.

Common Side Effects (Nausea, Digestive Changes)

Nausea

One of the most frequently reported side effects of prenatal vitamins is nausea. During pregnancy, many women are already dealing with morning sickness, and adding a prenatal supplement to the mix can sometimes amplify this feeling. Nausea can be especially common when taking a supplement that contains iron, an essential mineral for both mother and baby but one that can be rough on the stomach. Ritual Essential Prenatal has a delayed-release design to reduce this side effect, but a few women may still experience mild nausea.

Managing Nausea

If nausea strikes, there are a few steps you can take to make the experience more manageable:

1. Take with Food

While Ritual Prenatal doesn't require food for absorption, pairing it with a light meal or snack can help settle your stomach. Plain foods like crackers, toast, or applesauce are gentle on the digestive system and may help reduce queasiness.

2. Try Taking It in the Evening

If morning sickness is making it difficult to tolerate the prenatal in the early hours, consider taking it at night. Many women find that nausea subsides later in the day, making it easier to take the vitamin before bed when their stomachs are calmer.

3. Pair with Ginger or Peppermint Tea

Natural remedies like ginger or peppermint tea can help calm nausea. Sipping on a warm cup of ginger tea or keeping ginger chews on hand can provide immediate relief if you start to feel queasy.

Digestive Changes

The high nutrient density in a prenatal vitamin can sometimes lead to digestive changes, such as bloating, gas, or mild stomach discomfort. Iron, for example, is notorious for causing constipation in some people, while high levels of certain vitamins and minerals can affect the body's normal rhythm. Ritual Prenatal aims to alleviate these issues by using a form of iron that's easier on digestion, yet some users might still notice subtle changes.

Managing Digestive Changes

Here are a few tips to ease any digestive discomfort:

1. Stay Hydrated

Drinking enough water each day can make a significant difference in keeping digestion smooth. Aim for at least 8-10 glasses a day, especially if you're experiencing constipation. Hydration helps the body process nutrients more efficiently and can prevent sluggish digestion.

2. Increase Fiber Intake

A diet rich in fiber can help counteract any digestive slowdown caused by iron. Consider incorporating fiber-rich foods like whole grains, leafy greens, and fresh fruits into your meals to encourage regularity.

3. Move Your Body

Light exercise, like walking or stretching, can aid in digestion and help prevent discomfort. If you're feeling bloated or constipated, a short walk can get things moving and bring some relief.

4. Try Probiotic Foods

Foods like yogurt, kefir, sauerkraut, and kombucha can introduce beneficial bacteria to your digestive system, which may help balance out any disruption and reduce gas or bloating.

Rare but Possible Reactions

While Ritual Prenatal is carefully formulated to be safe and well-tolerated, rare but possible reactions can still occur. These are generally mild and include symptoms that might arise if you have sensitivities or an allergy to one of the ingredients. For example, although Ritual ensures its products are free from common allergens like gluten and soy, some women may experience reactions to specific ingredients like omega-3 or folate.

Potential Rare Reactions

1. Mild Allergic Reactions

Signs of a mild allergic reaction may include itching, hives, or mild swelling. If you notice these symptoms after taking the vitamin, it's a good idea to consult with a healthcare provider to assess whether you have an allergy to any of the ingredients.

2. Skin Changes

Occasionally, some people report minor skin reactions such as breakouts or slight rashes. These can sometimes be a result of an increased intake of specific nutrients, which may stimulate skin changes. If this happens, consider speaking with a healthcare provider or dermatologist to determine if your body needs time to adjust.

3. Headaches

High doses of certain vitamins, like B vitamins, can sometimes lead to headaches in sensitive individuals. If you experience headaches after starting the prenatal, this may be a sign to take it with a more substantial meal or to consult a healthcare professional to adjust the dosage.

Tips to Minimize Side Effects

In most cases, any side effects associated with taking Ritual Essential Prenatal Multivitamin can be managed with small adjustments. Here are some practical tips to help minimize discomfort and make your experience as comfortable as possible:

Tip 1: Establish a Routine

Your body often adapts better when it has a set rhythm. Try to take the vitamin at the same time each day, whether it's in the morning or at night. This helps your system anticipate and process the nutrients more efficiently, potentially reducing any side effects over time.

Tip 2: Start with a Lower Dosage

If you're sensitive to supplements, consider starting with just one capsule a day for the first week and then gradually increasing to the full dosage. This can give your body a gentler introduction to the new nutrient levels, reducing the chance of side effects. However, always consult with a healthcare provider before adjusting the dosage.

Tip 3: Pair with Anti-Nausea Strategies

As mentioned earlier, ginger and peppermint are great natural anti-nausea remedies. You could also keep snacks nearby if you feel a wave of nausea coming on after taking the vitamin. Simple, bland foods tend to settle the stomach quickly.

Tip 4: Adjust Your Diet

If you're taking a prenatal vitamin, your body is receiving an influx of nutrients that can sometimes throw off your usual balance. Adjust your diet to work in harmony with the supplement, adding more fiber-rich foods if you notice constipation or high-water-content foods if you feel dehydrated. Small dietary tweaks can make a big difference in managing side effects.

Tip 5: Talk to Your Healthcare Provider

If you experience any persistent or severe side effects, it's always best to speak with a healthcare provider. They may suggest taking the vitamin at a different time of day, adjusting your diet further, or switching to a different formulation if needed. Always prioritize your comfort and wellbeing, and never hesitate to seek advice when you need it.

Tip 6: Be Patient with the Adjustment Period

It's common for your body to need a few days or even a couple of weeks to adjust to a new prenatal vitamin. Minor side effects are often temporary as your system gets used to the additional nutrients. Patience and consistency can help you ease through this transition smoothly.

Taking Ritual Essential Prenatal Multivitamin is a powerful step toward supporting your pregnancy journey, but it's essential to listen to your body along the way. Side effects, if they occur, are usually manageable with small adjustments, and they often lessen as your body adapts to the new nutrient levels.

By following these practical tips, establishing a steady routine, and incorporating remedies for nausea or digestive issues, you can make the most of this supplement with minimal discomfort. As always, if you encounter side effects that feel unusual or persistent, reach out to your healthcare provider. Every woman's pregnancy journey is unique, and the key is to find a routine that best supports your body's.

CHAPTER 6; PRECAUTIONS AND CONTRAINDICATIONS

Prenatal vitamins like Ritual Essential Prenatal Multivitamin are carefully formulated to provide expectant mothers with the nutrients they need to support a healthy pregnancy. However, even the best prenatal supplement may not be suitable for everyone. Understanding who should avoid this product, potential interactions with medications or health conditions, and safety warnings during pregnancy is essential to ensuring both mother and baby are safe. This chapter will provide clear insights on precautions and contraindications, empowering you to make the most informed decision about using Ritual Essential Prenatal.

Who Should Avoid This Product

Individuals with Allergies to Certain Ingredients

Ritual Essential Prenatal Multivitamin is formulated with high-quality ingredients, but it may still contain elements that can trigger allergies in some individuals. This multivitamin is free from common allergens like soy, gluten, and dairy, but individuals with specific sensitivities or allergies should review the ingredient list thoroughly. For instance:

Wheat Allergy: Although Ritual products are processed to be gluten-free, they contain certain derivatives that may still cause reactions in highly sensitive individuals. If you have a known wheat allergy, it's essential to consult with a healthcare provider before use.

Fish Allergy: While Ritual's omega-3 source is derived from microalgae (making it vegan), individuals with extreme sensitivities should still verify with their healthcare provider, as microalgae production environments may pose potential sensitivities for those with fish or marine allergies.

Those with Pre-Existing Health Conditions

Not every supplement is appropriate for everyone, especially individuals managing specific health conditions. If you're dealing with any of the following conditions, consult your healthcare provider before starting this prenatal:

1. Kidney Disorders

People with certain kidney issues may need to limit their intake of specific nutrients, particularly those that the kidneys work to filter. Too much vitamin D or calcium can burden the kidneys, which may not be ideal for individuals with reduced kidney function.

2. Iron Overload Disorders (Hemochromatosis)

Ritual Prenatal includes iron, an essential mineral for many women during pregnancy. However, those with hemochromatosis or similar iron overload disorders should avoid iron supplements unless specifically directed by a healthcare provider, as excess iron can accumulate to harmful levels.

3. Blood Disorders and Clotting Conditions

If you have a condition that affects blood clotting, such as certain forms of hemophilia or a history of thrombotic events, you should discuss the safety of prenatal vitamins with a healthcare provider. Vitamins and minerals that influence blood properties, like iron and folate, may need to be carefully managed in these cases.

Individuals with Severe Nausea or Hyperemesis Gravidarum

For some women, pregnancy brings on severe nausea, including a condition known as hyperemesis gravidarum (HG), characterized by extreme, persistent nausea and vomiting. While Ritual Prenatal is designed to be gentle on the stomach with delayed-release technology, some women with HG may still find it challenging to take any supplement. In such cases, working closely with a healthcare provider can help you explore alternative ways to obtain the necessary nutrients, whether through smaller doses, liquid formulations, or alternative delivery methods.

Specific Interactions with Medications or Health Conditions

Medications That May Interact with Prenatal Vitamins

Some medications may interact with the nutrients in Ritual Essential Prenatal, impacting either the medication's effectiveness or the absorption of the vitamin itself. The following types of medications are worth noting:

1. Antacids and Acid Reducers
Medications like proton pump inhibitors (PPIs) and other antacids, commonly taken for heartburn, can reduce stomach acidity, which may in turn impact how well your body absorbs certain nutrients in the prenatal, such as calcium and iron. If you are on these medications, your healthcare provider may suggest alternative timing for taking your prenatal or recommend adjusting your diet to support nutrient absorption.

2. Blood Thinners

If you are prescribed anticoagulants like warfarin, the extra iron and vitamin K found in many prenatals may interfere with the medication's effectiveness. If you are taking blood thinners, discuss with your healthcare provider the safest approach to prenatal vitamins. They may advise adjustments in timing or even a specialized formulation with reduced vitamin K.

3. Thyroid Medications

Thyroid medications, such as levothyroxine, can interact with prenatal vitamins, particularly if they contain calcium and iron. These minerals can reduce the effectiveness of thyroid medication if taken at the same time. If you are taking thyroid medication, try to space your prenatal and thyroid medication doses by at least four hours for optimal effectiveness.

Health Conditions That Require Special Nutritional Considerations

Individuals with the following health conditions may need specific guidance when considering Ritual Essential Prenatal Multivitamin:

1. Diabetes or Insulin Resistance

While Ritual Prenatal is designed with balanced levels of nutrients, some women with diabetes or insulin resistance may need to monitor how the addition of specific nutrients influences blood sugar levels. Working with a healthcare provider can help you determine any adjustments needed in your nutrition plan.

2. Autoimmune Conditions

If you have an autoimmune condition, discuss with your healthcare provider which nutrients may be most beneficial or potentially detrimental to your condition. For instance, excess iron may sometimes aggravate symptoms in certain autoimmune diseases.

Important Safety Warnings During Pregnancy

When it comes to pregnancy, safety is paramount. Here are some safety considerations every expectant mother should keep in mind when taking prenatal vitamins:

Avoid Doubling Up on Vitamins

Sometimes, in the desire to be extra cautious, expectant mothers may be tempted to combine multiple vitamin supplements. However, taking more than the recommended dosage can increase the risk of vitamin toxicity, particularly with fat-soluble vitamins like A, D, E, and K, which can accumulate in the body if taken in excess. Ritual Prenatal is designed to meet daily nutrient needs for pregnancy; avoid taking additional multivitamins without consulting a healthcare provider.

Iron Intake Caution

Ritual Prenatal includes iron, which is critical for supporting blood health in both mother and baby.

However, excessive iron intake can lead to side effects like constipation, nausea, and, in extreme cases, iron toxicity. It's important not to take extra iron supplements unless advised by a healthcare provider.

Beware of Combining with Other Herbal Supplements

Some herbal supplements, while popular for supporting pregnancy symptoms, may not be safe to take with prenatal vitamins. Herbs like St. John's Wort or certain high-dose teas may interact with the nutrients in Ritual Essential Prenatal. Before combining herbal remedies with your prenatal, discuss it with a healthcare provider to ensure there are no risky interactions.

Storing Your Prenatal Vitamin Properly

Maintaining the integrity of your prenatal vitamin is essential for ensuring that each dose provides the right nutrients. Store Ritual Prenatal in a cool, dry place, away from direct sunlight. Additionally, keep it out of reach of children, as the high iron content can be harmful to young children if ingested accidentally. Choosing Ritual Essential Prenatal Multivitamin is an investment in your health and your baby's development. However, understanding who should avoid this product, potential medication interactions, and essential safety tips during pregnancy allows you to make an empowered choice with confidence. By consulting with a healthcare provider when necessary and staying informed, you can ensure that this prenatal vitamin serves as a safe and effective part of your pregnancy journey.

For expectant mothers, navigating the unique nutritional needs of pregnancy can be challenging, but Ritual Prenatal carefully chosen ingredients aim to offer peace of mind. Always remember that taking any supplement is a deeply personal decision, and what matters most is finding a safe, balanced solution that aligns with your body's needs, ultimately supporting the healthiest outcome for both you and your baby.

CHAPTER 7; EXPECTED BENEFITS OF RITUAL PRENATAL MULTIVITAMIN

Choosing the right prenatal vitamin is a crucial step in supporting both maternal and fetal health during pregnancy. Ritual Essential Prenatal Multivitamin offers a thoughtful blend of essential nutrients to support not only the mother's well-being but also the healthy development of the baby. Beyond pregnancy, its balanced formula can help ensure a strong nutritional foundation that carries into postpartum recovery and beyond. This chapter covers the expected benefits of Ritual Prenatal for the expectant mother, the developmental benefits for the baby, and the longer-term nutritional impacts.

Health Benefits for the Expectant Mother

Pregnancy brings about significant changes in a woman's body, increasing the demand for specific vitamins and minerals to support both maternal health and the baby's growth. Ritual Prenatal is designed with carefully selected ingredients to meet these increased needs, offering the following benefits for expectant mothers:

Supporting Energy Levels and Reducing Fatigue

Fatigue is a common experience during pregnancy, especially in the first and third trimesters. Ritual Prenatal provides iron, a critical component for blood health, which supports oxygen transport and helps reduce the risk of iron-deficiency anemia. Adequate iron intake can help expectant mothers maintain healthier energy levels, making it easier to keep up with the demands of pregnancy. In addition to iron, Ritual Prenatal includes B12 and other B vitamins, which play a key role in converting food into energy. These nutrients contribute to improved stamina and help reduce the feelings of exhaustion that can accompany pregnancy.

Enhancing Immune Support

During pregnancy, a woman's immune system becomes more sensitive, as it works to protect both the mother and the developing fetus. Ritual Prenatal contains vitamin D, an essential nutrient for immune health. Vitamin D helps regulate immune responses and, along with zinc, provides a vital layer of defense against common infections. A well-supported immune system can make a significant difference for expectant mothers, as even minor illnesses can feel more intense during pregnancy. By ensuring optimal levels of these nutrients, Ritual Prenatal aids in maintaining immune resilience during this critical period.

Maintaining Bone Health

Calcium is vital for bone health, and since pregnancy demands more calcium to support fetal development, it's important for expectant mothers to have enough available to meet their own needs as well. While Ritual Prenatal doesn't contain calcium, it includes vitamin D and magnesium, which help the body absorb and utilize calcium more effectively. Together, these nutrients contribute to the mother's bone health, helping reduce the risk of bone density loss that can sometimes occur during pregnancy.

Developmental Benefits for the Baby

The nutrients in Ritual Prenatal aren't just for the mother—they're carefully chosen to support the baby's growth and development in the womb. From brain formation to bone development, these vitamins and minerals are critical to giving the baby the best possible start in life.

Brain and Neural Development

One of the standout ingredients in Ritual Prenatal is choline, a nutrient critical for brain development and neural tube formation. Adequate choline intake supports healthy brain growth, helping lay the foundation for memory, learning, and emotional regulation later in life.

The inclusion of choline ensures that the mother is meeting the recommended amount, which many diets may lack. Additionally, folate (the natural form of folic acid) is essential for preventing neural tube defects, which are serious birth defects that affect the spine and brain. The folate in Ritual Prenatal is provided in its most absorbable form, methylated folate, ensuring that it's available to the baby for proper neural development.

Supporting Eye Development

Vitamin A, provided in Ritual Prenatal in the form of beta-carotene, plays a crucial role in the development of the baby's eyes. Proper vitamin A intake supports the formation of the retina and other eye structures, promoting healthy vision from birth. The beta-carotene in Ritual Prenatal is also safer than synthetic vitamin A, as it converts into the active form only as the body needs it, preventing the risk of vitamin A toxicity.

Healthy Bone and Skeletal Development

Magnesium and vitamin D are essential for the baby's skeletal growth. These nutrients work together to support bone mineralization, helping the baby develop strong bones and teeth. Calcium from the mother's diet is also essential for fetal bone growth, and the vitamin D and magnesium in Ritual Prenatal make it easier for the body to use calcium effectively. Proper skeletal development lays a foundation for lifelong bone health, reducing the risk of fractures and bone-related issues later in life.

Heart and Circulatory Health

Omega-3 DHA, derived from microalgae in Ritual Prenatal, is an essential fatty acid that supports the baby's cardiovascular development. DHA plays a critical role in forming the heart, blood vessels, and other circulatory structures. Studies show that sufficient intake of DHA during pregnancy can positively impact fetal heart health and may even support healthy blood pressure as the baby grows. Omega-3s are also beneficial for brain development, making DHA a double-duty nutrient that supports multiple facets of the baby's growth.

Long-Term Nutritional Impact Postpartum

After the baby arrives, maintaining a strong nutritional foundation is equally important as a mother transitions into the postpartum period. Ritual Prenatal can continue to provide several long-term benefits that support both the mother's health and her ability to care for her newborn.

Postpartum Recovery and Energy Support

The demands on a new mother's body don't stop after childbirth; in fact, they often increase as she recovers and adapts to the demands of caring for a newborn. The iron, B vitamins, and magnesium in Ritual Prenatal are particularly beneficial for supporting energy and vitality during this time. By replenishing iron lost during childbirth and providing key nutrients for energy, Ritual

Prenatal helps mothers feel more capable of meeting the physical and emotional demands of motherhood.

Support for Lactation

For mothers who choose to breastfeed, maintaining optimal nutrition remains essential. Certain nutrients, like vitamin D and omega-3 DHA, continue to play a significant role in supporting both the mother's and the baby's health through breast milk. DHA, in particular, can support the baby's brain and eye development through breastfeeding, providing a continuous benefit during this critical period of growth.

Bone Health and Hormonal Balance

Postpartum recovery can place additional stress on a mother's bones, especially if calcium stores were depleted during pregnancy. The vitamin D and magnesium in Ritual Prenatal support bone density and help regulate the hormones involved in bone health, reducing the risk of bone density loss and ensuring a smoother recovery. Hormonal balance is another aspect of postpartum health that benefits from proper nutrition. Nutrients like vitamin D, iron, and omega-3 DHA play supportive roles in mood regulation and mental health, which can help mothers manage the emotional shifts that come with the postpartum period. Ritual Essential Prenatal Multivitamin is more than just a prenatal supplement; it's a carefully crafted formula designed to support a mother's health through pregnancy, the baby's optimal growth and development, and the mother's recovery postpartum. By providing essential nutrients like folate, choline, omega-3 DHA, and vitamin D in their most absorbable forms, this prenatal vitamin helps set the stage for a healthier pregnancy and a strong foundation for both mother and baby. Investing in high-quality nutrition during pregnancy not only enhances the mother's health but also contributes to the baby's long-term well-being. Ritual Prenatal targeted formula addresses key areas of growth and development, ensuring that every capsule brings valuable benefits that support the journey of motherhood from start to finish.

CHAPTER 8; INTERACTIONS WITH OTHER SUPPLEMENTS AND MEDICATIONS

When it comes to prenatal vitamins, understanding how they interact with other supplements and medications is essential to maximizing benefits and minimizing potential risks. While Ritual Essential Prenatal Multivitamin is thoughtfully designed to support pregnancy with high-quality, well-researched nutrients, some interactions may arise if it's combined with other supplements or medications. This chapter provides an in-depth look into vitamins and minerals that may interact with Ritual Prenatal, guidance on combining it with other prenatal products, and warnings about certain medications and herbal supplements.

Vitamins and Minerals That May Interact

Prenatal vitamins pack in a host of nutrients, but taking additional supplements with similar ingredients can lead to excessive intake of certain vitamins and minerals. Knowing how these vitamins and minerals interact can help expectant mothers safely incorporate other supplements, if necessary, without unintended side effects.

Iron and Calcium

One key ingredient in Ritual Prenatal is iron, which is essential for oxygen transport and energy levels during pregnancy. However, calcium can hinder iron absorption when taken simultaneously, as both minerals compete for absorption in the intestines. If additional calcium is required, it's often recommended to take it separately from a prenatal vitamin to maximize iron absorption.

How to Handle This Interaction: For optimal benefits, take Ritual Prenatal at one time and any additional calcium supplement a few hours apart, ideally with a meal that doesn't contain iron-rich foods.

Vitamin D and Calcium

Vitamin D works synergistically with calcium, as it helps the body absorb and utilize calcium more effectively. However, taking high doses of calcium alongside a prenatal vitamin that includes vitamin D could increase the risk of calcium-related issues, such as kidney stones. The vitamin D in Ritual Prenatal is carefully balanced, so additional vitamin D or calcium should only be added to your regimen with the guidance of a healthcare provider.

How to Handle This Interaction: Ensure that any extra calcium or vitamin D supplement aligns with the levels in Ritual Prenatal and only add more if medically advised. If needed, your healthcare provider may recommend a lower or higher dose based on your individual needs.

Folate and Folic Acid

Ritual Prenatal contains folate, the natural form of vitamin B9, which is essential for preventing neural tube defects and promoting healthy fetal development. However, some prenatal supplements contain folic acid, the synthetic form of vitamin B9. It's essential to avoid taking excessive folic acid from additional supplements alongside Ritual Prenatal, as high levels of folic acid can mask symptoms of vitamin B12 deficiency.

How to Handle This Interaction: Avoid combining Ritual Prenatal with additional supplements containing folic acid unless specifically instructed by your healthcare provider. Ritual's use of methylated folate ensures effective absorption, eliminating the need for excessive folate intake.

Guidance on Combining with Other Prenatal Products

Many women wonder if they should be taking multiple prenatal products to "cover all bases" of nutrition.

However, combining multiple prenatal products can lead to overlapping ingredients, resulting in overconsumption of certain vitamins and minerals. Here's how to make the most of Ritual Prenatal alongside other prenatal essentials without overloading on nutrients.

Avoid Doubling Up on Multivitamins

If you're already taking Ritual Prenatal, adding another prenatal vitamin isn't recommended, as it can cause an intake of nutrients that exceed the recommended daily values, which can be harmful. Ritual Prenatal is designed to meet the nutritional needs of most pregnant women when paired with a balanced diet, so taking an additional prenatal isn't necessary.

How to Handle This Interaction: Stick to one high-quality prenatal vitamin to avoid doubling up on ingredients like iron, folate, and fat-soluble vitamins such as A, D, and E. If you feel you're missing a specific nutrient, consult your healthcare provider before adding a single-ingredient supplement to your routine.

Omega-3 and DHA Supplements

Ritual Prenatal already includes omega-3 DHA, derived from microalgae, to support fetal brain and eye development. If you're considering taking an additional omega-3 or DHA supplement, it's crucial to check the dosage, as excessive DHA could cause mild side effects like gastrointestinal discomfort or bleeding issues due to its blood-thinning properties.

How to Handle This Interaction: Since Ritual Prenatal already contains DHA, consult with a healthcare provider before adding any more omega-3 supplements In most cases, the included DHA is sufficient for prenatal needs, and adding more isn't necessary unless specifically recommended.

Adding Probiotics or Fiber

Some pregnant women experience digestive changes and turn to probiotics or fiber supplements to help. Generally, probiotics or fiber can be safely added to a prenatal regimen as they don't typically interact with vitamins or minerals. However, it's a good idea to ensure any added supplements don't contain excessive or unnecessary additives.

How to Handle This Interaction: If you're adding probiotics or fiber, check the ingredients list to ensure there's no overlap with Ritual Prenatal's components. Probiotics can be taken at any time, but fiber is best spaced out from Ritual Prenatal to avoid minor gastrointestinal side effects.

Medication and Herbal Supplement Warnings

Pregnancy can be a time when prescription medications, over-the-counter drugs, and herbal supplements are used more frequently to manage symptoms or preexisting conditions. However, combining these with prenatal vitamins can sometimes produce unintended effects. Here are the main categories to watch out for:

Blood-Thinning Medications

Some ingredients in prenatal vitamins, such as omega-3 DHA, may have mild blood-thinning effects. If you are on prescription blood thinners, including warfarin or aspirin, or if you are taking herbal supplements with blood-thinning properties (such as ginkgo biloba), it's important to monitor this with your healthcare provider.

How to Handle This Interaction: Inform your healthcare provider if you're taking any blood-thinning medications or supplements. They may recommend monitoring certain parameters or adjusting the dosage to balance the effects safely.

Thyroid Medications

Prenatal vitamins containing iron and calcium can interfere with the absorption of thyroid medications like levothyroxine. This means taking them simultaneously can reduce the efficacy of your thyroid medication, which is essential to manage during pregnancy.

How to Handle This Interaction: Take thyroid medication and Ritual Prenatal several hours apart to allow for proper absorption of each. Consult your doctor to create a balanced schedule that ensures maximum effectiveness of both.

Herbal Supplements (e.g., St. John's Wort, Ginseng)

Many herbal supplements have uncertain safety profiles during pregnancy and can interfere with prenatal vitamins or medications. For instance, St. John's Wort, often used for mood support, can reduce the effectiveness of certain medications, while ginseng may have stimulating effects that could impact maternal blood pressure.

How to Handle This Interaction: Avoid combining herbal supplements with Ritual Prenatal without consulting your healthcare provider. Stick to well-researched supplements if necessary, and be transparent with your provider about any herbal products you are using.

Over-the-Counter Medications

Common medications like antacids, which contain calcium or magnesium, can also interfere with iron absorption in prenatal vitamins. Antacids can be helpful for pregnancy-related heartburn but should be timed carefully when taken alongside Ritual Prenatal.

How to Handle This Interaction: If you need to take antacids, space them out by a few hours from your prenatal to ensure that iron absorption remains unaffected. Additionally, check with a healthcare professional if you are taking other over-the-counter medications to confirm there are no interactions with your prenatal routine. When using Ritual Essential Prenatal Multivitamin, understanding how it interacts with other supplements, medications, and herbal remedies can help you make safe, informed decisions for yourself and your baby. This prenatal vitamin is designed to be comprehensive, so there's rarely a need to add other multivitamins.

For single-ingredient supplements, ensure they don't overlap with Ritual's formula, and always consult a healthcare provider before introducing new products into your routine. By practicing careful timing and consulting with your healthcare provider, you can make the most of Ritual Prenatal to support a healthy, well-nourished pregnancy.

CHAPTER 9; STORAGE AND HANDLING OF RITUAL PRENATAL

Proper storage and handling of any supplement, especially prenatal vitamins, are essential to preserving its potency, quality, and safety. Ritual Essential Prenatal Multivitamin is formulated with high-quality ingredients, and how it's stored can make a big difference in how well these nutrients maintain their integrity over time. This chapter covers the ideal storage conditions, understanding the shelf-life and expiration details, and essential safe handling practices to help you get the best out of each capsule, ensuring it remains as effective and beneficial as intended.

Ideal Storage Conditions

Ritual Prenatal Multivitamin is meticulously crafted with nutrients that are designed to support both mother and baby. However, vitamins and supplements can be sensitive to environmental factors, especially heat, humidity, and light. When exposed to these conditions, vitamins may degrade faster, which can lead to reduced effectiveness.

Temperature

Temperature is one of the most crucial factors in supplement storage. Ideally, Ritual Prenatal should be stored in a cool, stable environment, away from direct sunlight and extreme temperatures. The recommended storage temperature is generally between 59-77°F (15-25°C), which is typical of indoor, room-temperature conditions. Storing your vitamins in a hot car, bathroom, or near a window can expose them to temperature fluctuations that may break down delicate nutrients over time.

Pro Tip: Keep your Ritual Prenatal bottle in a dark, cool cabinet or pantry. If you live in a particularly hot climate, consider finding the coolest spot in your home for storage. Avoid placing the bottle in the fridge, as the moisture could lead to clumping and reduced capsule quality.

Humidity

Humidity is another important environmental factor, as excess moisture can cause supplements to clump, degrade, or even develop mold over time. For example, storing supplements in a bathroom is generally discouraged because showers and baths can create a humid environment. Additionally, humidity can interact with the capsule's shell, potentially making it sticky or causing it to deteriorate more quickly.

Pro Tip: Always keep the cap tightly closed after each use to prevent moisture from entering the bottle. If you're taking your vitamins with a drink, pour the desired number of capsules into your hand first, rather than directly over a drink, to prevent accidental moisture exposure.

Light Exposure

Light, particularly UV light from the sun, can degrade the potency of certain vitamins, especially those in transparent or light-colored containers. Ritual's opaque bottle is designed to block light exposure, providing an added layer of protection for the vitamins inside. However, it's still a good practice to store the bottle in a dark place to minimize light exposure further.

Pro Tip: A kitchen drawer or pantry shelf makes a great storage location, as both block out natural light and keep the vitamins safe. Avoid leaving the bottle on a countertop where it may be exposed to direct sunlight during the day.

Shelf-Life and Expiration Details

All supplements come with an expiration date, and Ritual Prenatal is no exception. The expiration date is an important guide, as it reflects the period during which the product is guaranteed to maintain its potency and safety under recommended storage conditions.

Understanding Expiration Dates

The expiration date printed on the bottle indicates the point after which the vitamins may begin to lose their efficacy. Nutrients such as vitamins and minerals naturally degrade over time, and while taking expired vitamins is generally not harmful, it's not ideal because they may no longer provide the full nutritional support needed during pregnancy.

Pro Tip: Check the expiration date when you receive a new bottle, and try to finish the bottle before this date. Typically, prenatal vitamins are consumed daily, so it's easy to stay on schedule if you're taking them as recommended.

Signs of Vitamin Degradation

Sometimes, even before the expiration date, supplements can show signs of degradation if they've been exposed to poor storage conditions. Here are a few things to look out for:

Color Change: A change in the color of the capsule or its contents can be a sign that the vitamins have been exposed to heat, light, or moisture.

Texture Alterations: Clumping, stickiness, or an unusual texture on the surface of the capsule could indicate excess moisture.

Smell: If the capsules develop an unusual or off-putting smell, it could mean that they're no longer fresh.

If you notice any of these changes, it's best to consult the manufacturer or replace the bottle, especially if it's close to or past its expiration date.

Pro Tip: Write the date you open a new bottle on the label. Most vitamins retain peak potency for a set duration after opening, usually around three to six months, so keeping track can help ensure you're consuming them within their optimal period.

Safe Handling Practices

In addition to proper storage, handling your Ritual Prenatal vitamins with care is important to preserve their quality. Supplements may seem stable, but they're actually sensitive to everyday mishandling that can compromise their effectiveness. Here's how to keep them safe:

Avoid Transferring to Other Containers

While it may be tempting to move your prenatal vitamins into a pill organizer or another container, it's generally best to keep them in their original bottle. The Ritual packaging is specifically designed to protect the vitamins from light, air, and moisture. Transferring them to a different container may inadvertently expose them to these elements.

Pro Tip: If you need to carry a small portion of your vitamins on the go, consider purchasing a travel-sized version or small pill case and refill it only as needed. Be sure to store it in a similar environment as the original bottle when possible.

Handle Capsules with Dry Hands

Moisture from wet or damp hands can contribute to the degradation of vitamins, especially when moisture-sensitive ingredients are involved. If your hands are wet when you reach into the bottle, it can transfer moisture to the remaining capsules, potentially affecting their quality.

Pro Tip: Dry your hands completely before opening the bottle. Another option is to pour the vitamins directly into the bottle cap or a small cup instead of handling them directly, which helps keep the remaining capsules dry and fresh.

Close the Cap Tightly After Each Use

It might seem like a small detail, but closing the cap tightly after each use can significantly impact the vitamins' freshness. The cap acts as a barrier, keeping out air and moisture. Leaving the bottle slightly open, even for a few hours, can allow air to seep in, which can contribute to the oxidation of certain nutrients.

Pro Tip: Make it a habit to securely close the bottle every time you finish using it. By simply ensuring a tight seal, you're helping protect the nutrients inside from unnecessary exposure.

Avoid Taking Supplements in Moist Environments

Many people have a routine of taking their vitamins in the bathroom or kitchen, where they keep water or juice readily available. However, the humidity from hot showers or cooking can impact the quality of the vitamins over time. By choosing a drier, cooler spot to store and take them, you're supporting a longer shelf-life and higher potency.

Pro Tip: Consider keeping a small bottle of water in your usual vitamin storage spot, so you don't have to transport the bottle to the bathroom or kitchen.

By following these simple storage and handling practices, you can protect the quality and potency of your Ritual Prenatal Multivitamin. This supplement is a valuable ally during pregnancy, designed with carefully chosen ingredients and technology to support you and your baby. Ensuring it's stored in optimal conditions allows you to receive its full benefits with each capsule, giving you peace of mind that you're nourishing your body and supporting your baby's development effectively. The right environment — cool, dry, and dark — combined with mindful handling will keep your Ritual Prenatal as fresh and potent as the day you opened it. Remember, small steps in caring for your vitamins translate to big steps in supporting your health and wellness journey.

CHAPTER 10; FREQUENTLY ASKED QUESTIONS

When it comes to taking prenatal vitamins, especially one as popular and well-regarded as Ritual Essential Prenatal Multivitamin, it's common for expectant mothers to have questions. This chapter aims to address the most frequently asked questions surrounding this supplement, clarifying common concerns, offering tips for optimal results, and providing answers tailored to specific scenarios that many women face during pregnancy. With clear and comprehensive guidance, this section will help you feel confident and informed in your prenatal journey.

Common Concerns Addressed

1. Is it necessary to take a prenatal vitamin?

Many women wonder whether a prenatal vitamin is necessary during pregnancy, especially if they believe they are eating a balanced diet. While a well-rounded diet is essential for both mother and baby, prenatal vitamins are specifically formulated to fill nutritional gaps. They contain higher levels of certain nutrients, such as folate and iron, which are crucial during pregnancy. These nutrients support fetal development and help prevent birth defects, making prenatal vitamins an important addition to a healthy lifestyle.

2. What is the difference between prenatal vitamins and regular multivitamins?

Prenatal vitamins differ from standard multivitamins in several ways. They are specifically designed to meet the nutritional needs of pregnant women, providing essential nutrients in amounts that support fetal growth and development. For instance, prenatal vitamins typically contain increased levels of folate, iron, and DHA, which may not be present in regular multivitamins at the necessary levels for pregnancy. Therefore, it's important to choose a prenatal vitamin that aligns with your specific health needs during this critical time.

3. Are there any allergens in Ritual Prenatal?

Ritual Prenatal Multivitamin is formulated to be free from common allergens such as gluten, dairy, and nuts. However, it's always advisable to check the product label for specific allergen information. If you have allergies or intolerances, consult with your healthcare provider before starting any new supplement to ensure it's safe for you.

Tips for Optimal Results and Use

1. Consistency is Key

One of the most effective ways to ensure you're getting the benefits of Ritual Prenatal is to take it consistently. Establishing a daily routine can help you remember to take your vitamins. Whether it's first thing in the morning with breakfast or right before bed, find a time that works for you and stick to it. Setting reminders on your phone or using a pill organizer can also be helpful.

2. Pair with Food for Better Absorption

Taking your prenatal vitamins with food can enhance absorption and minimize any potential digestive discomfort. Foods rich in healthy fats, such as avocados or nuts, can help your body better absorb fat-soluble vitamins (like A, D, E, and K) found in the multivitamin. Aim to take your Ritual Prenatal with a meal that includes some fat for optimal results.

3. Stay Hydrated

Adequate hydration is crucial, especially during pregnancy. Drinking plenty of water not only supports your overall health but also aids in digestion, helping your body absorb the nutrients from the multivitamin effectively. Aim to drink at least eight glasses of water a day to stay well-hydrated.

4. Monitor Your Body's Response

Pay attention to how your body reacts after taking the Ritual Prenatal Multivitamin. If you experience any unusual side effects or discomfort, consider consulting your healthcare provider. They can provide guidance on whether to adjust your dosage or suggest alternative supplements if necessary.

Answers to User-Specific Scenarios

1. What should I do if I forget to take a dose?

If you forget to take a dose of your Ritual Prenatal, don't panic. Simply take it as soon as you remember. However, if it's close to the time for your next dose, skip the missed one and continue with your regular schedule. Never double up on doses to make up for a missed one, as this can lead to excessive intake of certain nutrients.

2. Can I take Ritual Prenatal with other supplements?

If you're taking other supplements, it's essential to check for overlapping nutrients, particularly iron, calcium, and vitamin D. Too much of certain vitamins and minerals can lead to adverse effects. Discussing your supplement regimen with your healthcare provider ensures you're not exceeding recommended levels and that all supplements work together effectively.

3. What if I have dietary restrictions?

For those with dietary restrictions—such as vegans or vegetarians—Ritual Prenatal is an excellent option as it is free from animal products and designed to meet the nutritional needs of all women, regardless of their dietary choices. However, if you have specific restrictions or needs, consult your healthcare provider for tailored advice and additional supplementation if necessary.

4. How do I know if the prenatal vitamin is working?

It may not always be obvious if a prenatal vitamin is "working," as many benefits occur internally and are not immediately visible. However, you may notice improvements in your energy levels, hair health, and overall well-being. Regular prenatal check-ups will also help assess your nutritional status and ensure that both you and your baby are thriving. Your healthcare provider can monitor your blood levels of essential nutrients and provide guidance based on those results.

5. Is it safe to continue taking Ritual Prenatal while breastfeeding?

Many women choose to continue taking prenatal vitamins while breastfeeding to support their nutritional needs and maintain milk quality. However, the specific nutrient requirements may change postpartum. It's essential to consult with your healthcare provider to determine if you should continue with the prenatal multivitamin or switch to a postnatal supplement that may better suit your needs during breastfeeding.

Navigating the world of prenatal vitamins can feel overwhelming, but understanding your concerns, knowing the best practices for optimal use, and having answers to common scenarios can empower you during this journey. Ritual Essential Prenatal Multivitamin is designed to support you and your growing baby, providing the necessary nutrients to foster a healthy pregnancy. By incorporating these tips and addressing your specific needs, you can maximize the benefits of your prenatal vitamin and embark on this beautiful journey with confidence. Always consult with your healthcare provider if you have any doubts or require personalized guidance, ensuring that your prenatal experience is as healthy and positive as possible.

CONCLUSION

As you embark on the incredible journey of motherhood, every step you take is crucial for both you and your growing baby. The choices you make during this time can have lasting impacts on your health and the health of your child. One of the most significant decisions you can make is to prioritize your nutritional intake, and incorporating Ritual Essential Prenatal Multivitamin into your daily routine is a powerful way to do just that.

The importance of prenatal vitamins cannot be overstated. They are designed to complement your diet, ensuring that you receive the essential nutrients necessary for a healthy pregnancy. Ritual Prenatal Multivitamin stands out in the crowded supplement market due to its carefully curated formula that specifically targets the needs of expectant mothers. By combining vital nutrients such as folate and choline, Ritual supports not only your health but also the development of your baby.

At the heart of Ritual Prenatal Multivitamin is a commitment to providing the highest quality nutrients. Folate, for instance, plays a critical role in preventing neural tube defects and supporting fetal growth. Meanwhile, choline is essential for brain development and can help improve cognitive function in infants. These ingredients reflect a science-based approach to prenatal nutrition, recognizing that each nutrient serves a unique purpose in the complex tapestry of pregnancy.

Moreover, the product is free from common allergens, making it accessible to a broad range of women. This inclusivity is vital during a time when dietary restrictions may become necessary. Ritual ensures that you don't have to compromise on quality or effectiveness, even if you have specific dietary needs. Ritual's commitment to transparency and quality extends beyond the ingredients themselves. With the innovative delayed-release capsule design, you can be assured that the nutrients are absorbed efficiently, reducing the chances of digestive discomfort—a common concern during pregnancy.

The incorporation of lemon essence flavor tabs also makes the experience of taking your vitamins more pleasant, helping to mask any undesirable tastes without added sugars. In a world where time is often a luxury, the simplicity and convenience of Ritual's subscription model ensure that you never have to worry about running out of essential vitamins. You can adjust your delivery schedule to fit your lifestyle, making it easier than ever to maintain your health regimen.

Despite the many benefits, it's essential to recognize that no supplement is without its considerations. As discussed in previous chapters, potential side effects such as nausea and digestive changes can occur. However, being informed allows you to take proactive steps to mitigate these issues. For example, taking your vitamins with food or ensuring you're well-hydrated can make a significant difference in how your body reacts. Moreover, if you have specific health conditions or are taking other medications, it's crucial to consult with your healthcare provider. They can offer personalized guidance that considers your unique health profile, ensuring you get the most out of your prenatal regimen. The benefits of taking Ritual Essential Prenatal Multivitamin extend beyond the pregnancy period. Adequate nutrition during pregnancy can lay the foundation for your child's health in the years to come. Studies have shown that maternal nutrition plays a pivotal role in a child's long-term development, influencing everything from cognitive function to physical health.

By prioritizing your nutrition now, you are not only caring for yourself but also investing in your child's future. After childbirth, many women continue to seek ways to support their health, especially during the postpartum phase when demands can be high. Ritual offers a range of products tailored to this new stage of life, ensuring that your nutritional needs are met as you navigate the challenges and joys of motherhood. Another noteworthy aspect of choosing Ritual is the sense of community that comes with it. Many women find comfort in knowing they are not alone in their experiences.

Ritual fosters a supportive environment where expectant mothers can share their journeys, seek advice, and find encouragement from others who are on similar paths. This community aspect is invaluable during a time that can be filled with uncertainty and questions. Ultimately, the choice to take Ritual Essential Prenatal Multivitamin is more than just a health decision; it's an empowering step toward embracing motherhood with confidence.

By equipping yourself with the right nutrients, you are setting the stage for a healthier pregnancy and a brighter future for your child. As you move forward on this journey, remember that taking care of yourself is just as important as taking care of your baby. Every small step you take toward better nutrition and health contributes to a holistic approach to motherhood. Embrace this time with intention, curiosity, and care. In conclusion, Ritual Essential Prenatal Multivitamin is a thoughtfully designed supplement that can play a pivotal role in your pregnancy journey. With its commitment to quality ingredients, innovative formulation, and supportive community, Ritual empowers you to make informed choices about your health. As you navigate the beautiful, complex, and transformative experience of pregnancy, know that you are not only nurturing your own well-being but also fostering the health and happiness of the new life you are bringing into the world. So, as you stand at this exciting crossroads, take a deep breath and embrace the journey ahead. You are equipped with knowledge, support, and the right tools to ensure a vibrant, healthy pregnancy. Here's to the incredible adventure of motherhood, one step at a time!

www.ingramcontent.com/pod-product-compliance
Lightning Source LLC
Chambersburg PA
CBHW070424240526
45472CB00020B/1183